POSITIVE
PREGNANCY AFFIRMATIONS

POSITIVE
PREGNANCY AFFIRMATIONS

M NGAIHLIAN

ISBN: 9798865069737
Imprint: Independently published

This book is dedicated to You.
So, here is to you – Live your life to your full potential
as a wonderful mother.

Books By M Ngaihlian:

1. Living Beyond Regrets
2. What The Heck! Do It Anyway!
3. Living With Purpose And No Regrets
4. Does God Care About Me?
5. 120 Memory Verses For Kids
6. 3250+ Bible Verses For Every Day & Situation
7. Important Questions To Ask Yourself
8. Just Because You
9. I Am Affirmation Bible Verses For Girls
10. I Am Affirmation Bible Verses For Boys
11. I Am Affirmation Bible Verses For Women
12. I Am Affirmation Bible Verses For Men
13. Badass Positive Affirmations For Women
14. Badass Positive Affirmations For Men
15. Badass Positive Affirmations For Dads
16. Badass Positive Affirmations For Entrepreneurs
17. Badass Affirmations For Moms

INTRODUCTION

From the moment those two lines show up on the test, life suddenly takes on a whole new meaning. It's like being handed a one-way ticket to the wildest, most heartwarming journey you'll ever embark upon. From the cravings that make you question your taste buds to the magical sensation of feeling that first fluttery kick, every moment is a chapter in its own right.

From the endless debates on nursery themes to the hilarious, often nerve-wracking experience of picking the perfect name, it's a whirlwind of emotions. Then comes the big day, the labor of love that brings your tiny miracle into the world, instantly making all the pain and discomfort worthwhile. During those moments, you will find yourself speaking positive affirmations to you and your baby.

THE POWER OF POSITIVE AFFIRMATIONS

Affirmations are not mere self-talk or words. They tap into the intricate workings of your brain and your subconscious mind. When you consistently repeat positive affirmations, you are, in essence, rewiring your thought patterns. Your brain responds to these repetitive messages by creating new neural pathways, reinforcing positive beliefs, and challenging negative ones - unlocking your full potential and reshaping your life. They hold the power to transform your mindset, boost your self-confidence, and lead you on a path to personal growth and fulfillment during your pregnancy and your journey into motherhood.

Studies in neuroscience have shown that affirmations can stimulate the brain's reward centers, releasing dopamine—a neurotransmitter associated with pleasure and motivation. This creates a positive feedback loop, making you more likely to continue the affirmations and embrace the associated beliefs.

THE PSYCHOLOGY OF AFFIRMATIONS

Affirmations work because they operate on fundamental psychological principles. Here's how they can impact your mental and emotional well-being:

Boosting Self-Esteem:
Affirmations help counteract self-doubt and negative self-perception. By repeating positive statements about yourself, you gradually boost your self-esteem and self-worth.

Changing Negative Beliefs:
Often, we hold limiting beliefs about our capabilities or self-worth. Affirmations challenge these beliefs and encourage a more empowering perspective.

Shifting Focus:
Negative thoughts can dominate your mind and perpetuate a cycle of pessimism. Affirmations redirect your focus toward positive possibilities and opportunities.

Increasing Resilience:
Regular use of affirmations builds emotional resilience. You become better equipped to handle challenges, setbacks, and stress with a positive outlook.

Cultivating a Growth Mindset:
Affirmations foster a growth mindset—a belief that your abilities and intelligence can be developed through effort and learning. This mindset drives you to seek self-improvement.

HOW TO MANIFEST YOUR AFFIRMATIONS

Making affirmations work effectively involves more than just repeating positive statements but requires a strategic and mindful approach. To harness the power of positive affirmations effectively, consider these practical strategies:

Set Clear Goals:
Begin with a clear understanding of what you want to achieve. Define your goals and intentions. Affirmations are most powerful when they are aligned with specific objectives.

Be Specific And Customised Your Affirmations:
Tailor your positive affirmations to your goals and desires that resonate with your goals and values. Ensure they are positive, present tense, and achievable. Focus on specific areas of your life or qualities you want to improve. Personalize them so they resonate deeply with your aspirations. For instance, if you're aiming for a promotion, your affirmation could be, *"I am highly capable and deserving of the promotion I seek."*

Use Present Tense:
Phrase your affirmations in the present tense as if you're already experiencing the desired outcome. For example, instead of saying, *"I will be successful,"* say, *"I am successful."* This makes them more effective because your brain processes them as current reality.

Repeat Consistently:

Consistency is key. Incorporate affirmations into your daily routine—morning, noon, and night—to reinforce positive beliefs. To reap the benefits, repetition is vital. Make affirmations a daily ritual, just like brushing your teeth. Over time, they'll become a natural part of your thinking.

Believe in Them:

To make affirmations work, you must genuinely believe in them. It's not enough to just recite affirmations. You have to believe in what you're saying. If you don't, your subconscious mind won't buy it, and the magic won't happen. If you encounter resistance or skepticism, address those doubts.

Use Emotion and Visualization:

As you repeat affirmations, engage your emotions and imagination. Feel the emotions associated with the affirmations. While saying your affirmations, visualize yourself living the reality described in your affirmations. This adds a powerful dimension to their effectiveness.

Combine with Action:

While affirmations can influence your mindset, they work best when combined with action. Take steps, no matter how small, toward your goals. Action reinforces belief in your affirmations.

Eliminate Negative Self-Talk:

Pay attention to your inner dialogue and replace self-criticism with affirmations. When you catch yourself thinking negatively, counteract it with a positive affirmation.

Practice Patience:

Positive changes take time. Be patient with yourself. It may take weeks or even months to see significant results. Trust the process and remain committed.

Journal Your Progress:
Keep a journal to record your experiences and observations. Track any shifts in your mindset, behavior, or circumstances. Documenting your progress helps reinforce the effectiveness of affirmations.

Surround Yourself with Positivity:
Create an environment that supports your affirmations. Surround yourself with positive people, motivational quotes, and images that align with your goals.

Stay Open to Opportunities And Adapt:
Be receptive to opportunities that align with your affirmations. Act on these opportunities when they arise. Affirmations can guide your actions and decisions. As you make progress, revisit your affirmations regularly. Adjust them to reflect your evolving goals and beliefs. Growth and change are natural, so adapt your affirmations accordingly.

Seek Accountability and Support:
Share your affirmations and goals with a trusted friend, mentor, or coach. They can provide support, and encouragement, and hold you accountable.

Live the Affirmations:
Ultimately, affirmations work when you integrate their messages into your daily life. Let them guide your actions, decisions, and interactions. Live as if you've already embraced the positive beliefs they convey.

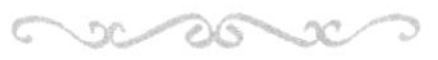

HOW TO USE THIS BOOK

1. Start with an Open Mind

Before you dive into the affirmations, approach this book with an open mind. Be willing to explore new ideas, challenge your existing beliefs, and embrace the potential for positive change in your life.

2. Set Clear Intentions

Begin by setting clear intentions for what you hope to achieve by using this book. What areas of your life do you want to improve? What specific goals do you want to work towards? Having a clear purpose will guide your journey.

3. Daily Affirmation Practice

The heart of this book lies in its affirmations. Each affirmation is a statement of empowerment, designed to reshape your mindset and boost your confidence. Incorporate these affirmations into your daily routine.

Morning Routine: Start your day by reading and reflecting on one or more affirmations. This will set a positive tone for the day ahead.

Throughout the Day: Carry a few affirmations with you on a small card or note in your pocket or wallet. Whenever you have a moment, revisit these affirmations to reinforce their messages.

Before Bed: End your day by revisiting the affirmations. Reflect on your experiences and how the affirmations impacted your thoughts and actions during the day.

4. Visualization

As you read and recite the affirmations, take a moment to visualize the positive outcomes they describe. Imagine yourself living the life you desire, achieving your goals, and embodying the qualities mentioned in the affirmations. Visualization adds depth and emotional connection to the process.

5. Journaling

Consider keeping a journal to record your experiences and reflections as you work with the affirmations. Write down any shifts in your mindset, any positive changes in your behavior, and any challenges you encounter. Journaling provides a valuable record of your progress.

6. Be Consistent

Consistency is crucial for the effectiveness of affirmations. Make a commitment to practice daily, even on days when you might not feel your best. Over time, the affirmations will become ingrained in your thinking.

7. Adapt and Customize

Feel free to adapt the affirmations to your specific goals and needs. You can modify them to make them more personal and relevant to your life. The key is to make them resonate with you on a deep level.

Affirmations are not just words but the embodiment of your inner potential. As you embrace their power, you will unlock the incredible capacity within you to create the life you desire—one empowered belief at a time. It's time to transform your mind and, in doing so, transform your life.

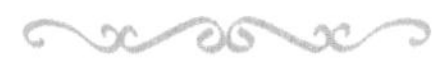

1

"I AM READY AND EXCITED TO EMBRACE THE JOYS AND CHALLENGES OF MOTHERHOOD"

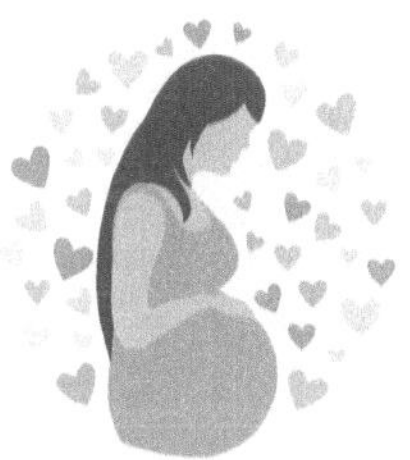

Embrace the journey of motherhood with readiness and enthusiasm. Approach the joys and challenges that come with raising a child with an open heart and a sense of adventure. Embrace the lessons and growth that accompany this transformative experience, knowing that every moment spent with your child is a precious gift that enriches your life in immeasurable ways.

2

"I AM GRATEFUL FOR THE PRIVILEGE OF BRINGING A NEW LIFE INTO THIS WORLD"

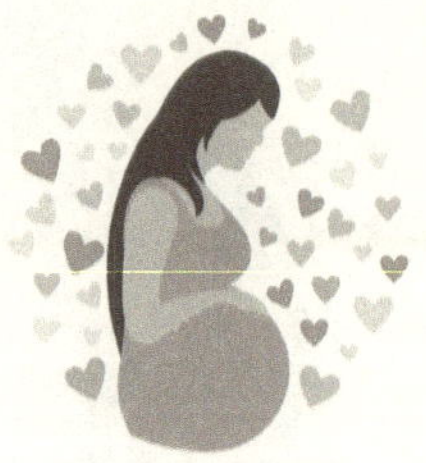

Express deep gratitude for the privilege and honor of bringing a new life into the world. Recognize the profound responsibility and joy that come with the role of motherhood, appreciating the transformative impact it has on your life. Cultivate a sense of appreciation and humility, knowing that the journey of motherhood is a sacred gift that is filled with love and purpose.

3

"MY BABY IS A GIFT, AND I AM HONORED TO BE CHOSEN AS A MOTHER"

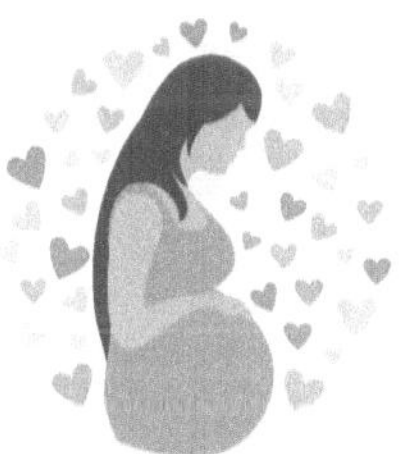

Embrace the profound honor of being chosen as the mother of your baby. Recognize the gift that your baby represents in your life, bringing boundless love and purpose into your world. Cherish the privilege of nurturing and guiding your child, knowing that it is a remarkable and sacred responsibility that you hold with grace and gratitude.

4

"MY BABY IS A MIRACLE, AND I AM BLESSED TO BE A PART OF THIS MIRACLE"

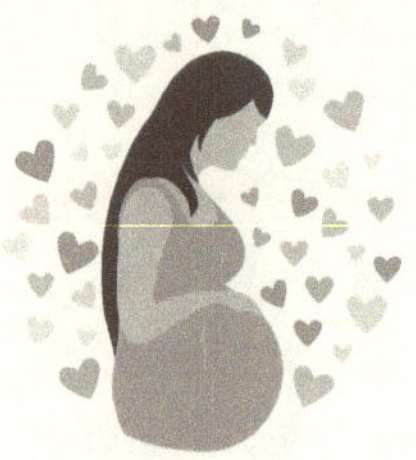

Embrace the profound miracle of life that is growing within you. Recognize the sacredness and wonder of this experience, knowing that you have been chosen to play a pivotal role in the creation of a new life. Appreciate the blessing of being a part of this miraculous journey, and let the awe and reverence you feel enrich your connection with your baby.

5

"MY BABY IS SURROUNDED BY LOVE AND POSITIVITY FROM THE MOMENT OF CONCEPTION"

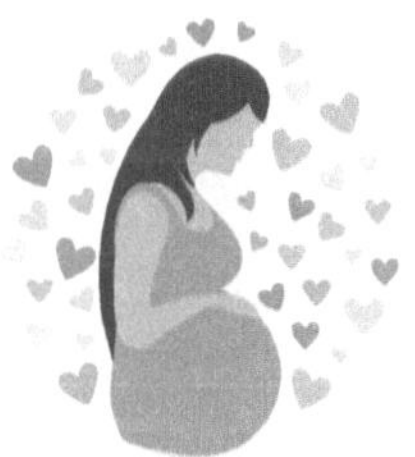

Envision your baby being surrounded by an abundance of love and positivity from the very beginning. Fill your thoughts and intentions with love, knowing that it reaches your baby even before they are born. Cultivate an atmosphere of positivity and joy, creating a nurturing environment that supports your baby's development and growth, both physically and emotionally.

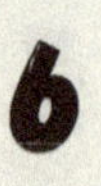

"MY BODY IS PERFECTLY DESIGNED TO NURTURE AND SUSTAIN NEW LIFE"

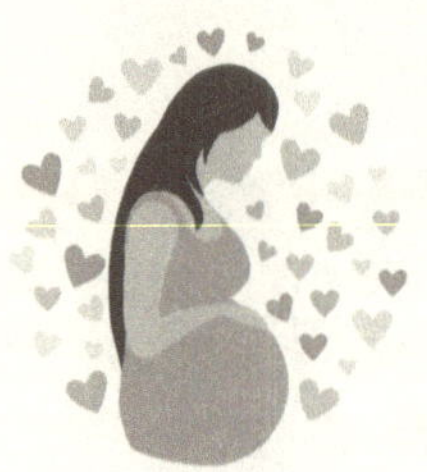

Recognize the perfection and intricacy of your body's design, especially when it comes to nurturing and sustaining new life. Acknowledge the physiological and emotional changes that occur during pregnancy as a testament to the remarkable capabilities of your body. Embrace the innate wisdom that your body possesses, knowing that it is equipped to provide the optimal conditions for your baby's growth and development.

7

"I AM CREATING A SAFE AND NURTURING SPACE FOR MY BABY"

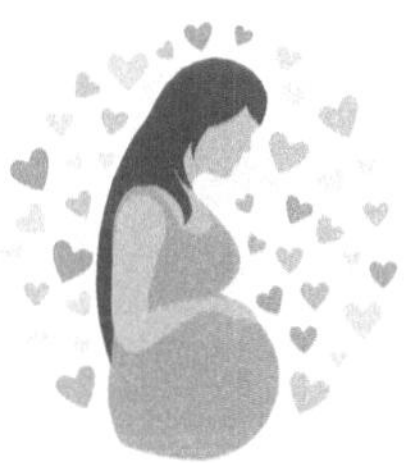

Your body is not just a home for you but a sanctuary for your growing baby. Every thought and action you take contributes to the environment your baby is experiencing. By surrounding yourself with positivity and love, you are fostering a nurturing space that will shape your baby's earliest experiences.

8

"I AM EMBRACING THE CHANGES IN MY BODY AS A BEAUTIFUL PART OF THIS PROCESS"

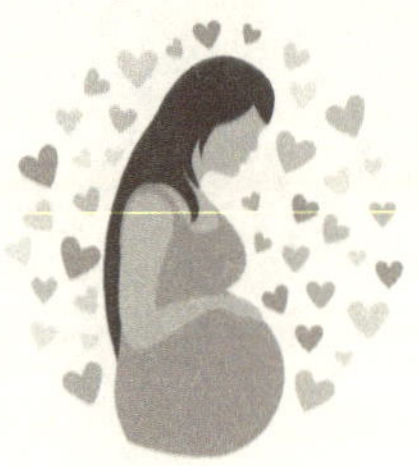

Embrace the changes in your body as a natural and beautiful part of the pregnancy journey. Appreciate the physical transformations as a testament to the incredible process of bringing new life into the world. Embrace the beauty of these changes, knowing that they signify the wondrous and transformative experience of motherhood.

9

"MY BODY IS CAPABLE AND STRONG, DESIGNED FOR THIS JOURNEY"

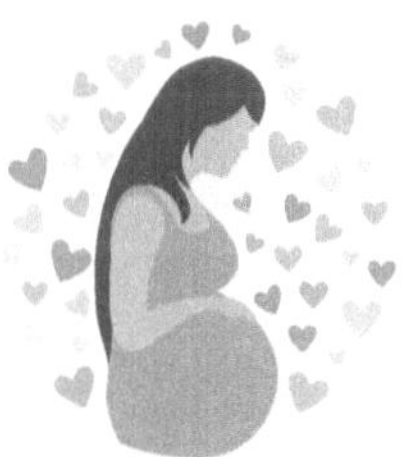

Trust in the inherent power and resilience of your body. It has been intricately designed to carry and nurture life. Acknowledge the incredible strength and adaptability it possesses to accommodate the changes necessary for the growth and development of your baby. You are a vessel of life, and your body is equipped for this miraculous journey.

10

"I TRUST MY BODY TO KNOW HOW TO GROW AND BIRTH MY BABY"

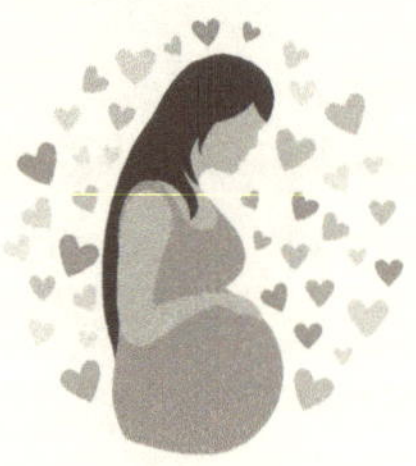

Believe in the innate wisdom of your body. It has an inherent intelligence that knows how to nurture and bring forth life. Trust in the process and allow your body to guide you through the various stages of pregnancy and childbirth. Know that it knows how to carry and birth your baby with grace and strength.

11

"MY BODY IS AN INCREDIBLE VESSEL, NURTURING AND PROTECTING MY BABY"

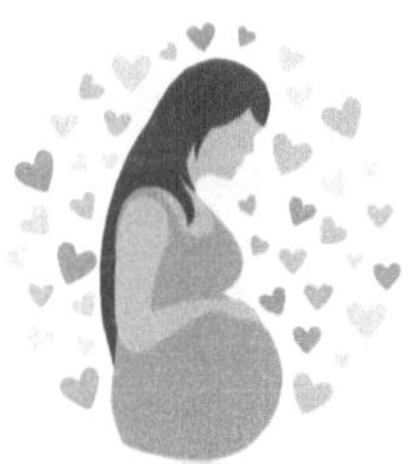

Recognize the remarkable role that your body plays in nurturing and protecting your growing baby. Appreciate the intricate processes and mechanisms that safeguard and support your baby's development. Trust in the innate ability of your body to create an optimal environment for your baby's growth and well-being.

12

"MY BODY IS A MIRACULOUS VESSEL, BRINGING FORTH NEW LIFE INTO THE WORLD"

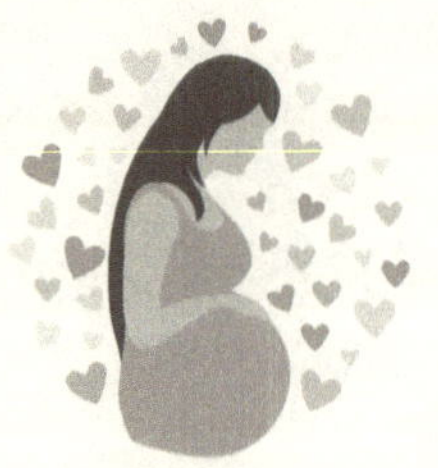

Recognize the miraculous nature of your body as it prepares to bring forth new life. Appreciate the intricacies and complexities that enable you to nurture and sustain your growing baby. Honor the sacredness of your body as it undergoes profound changes, acknowledging its remarkable ability to create and nurture life with grace and resilience.

13

"EACH DAY, MY BABY IS GROWING IN HEALTH AND STRENGTH"

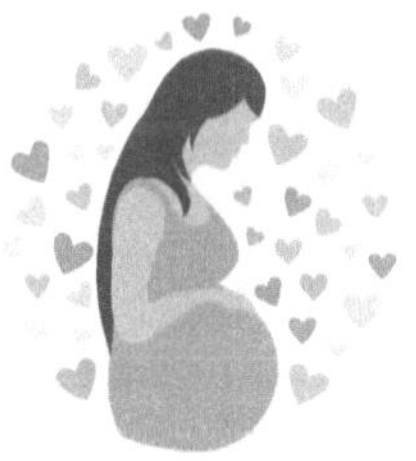

Visualize the profound miracle of life unfolding within you. With each passing day, your baby is gaining strength and vitality, supported by the nourishment and care you provide. Embrace the knowledge that your body is nurturing a healthy and robust life, laying the foundation for a strong and vibrant future.

14

"I AM SURROUNDED BY LOVE AND SUPPORT DURING THIS TIME"

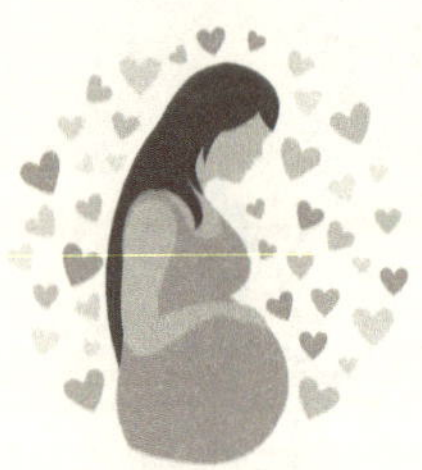

Feel the warmth of the love and support that envelops you during this special journey. Draw strength from the care and affection of your loved ones, who are there to uplift and encourage you every step of the way. Embrace the nurturing community around you, knowing that you are not alone on this path.

15

"I AM EMBRACING THE CHANGES IN MY BODY WITH GRACE AND ACCEPTANCE"

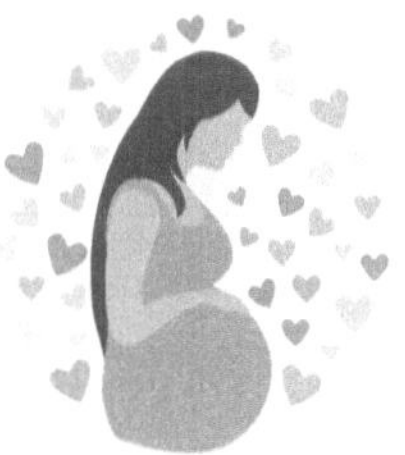

Honor the changes that your body is undergoing as a testament to the miracle of life within you. Embrace these changes with a sense of grace and acceptance, acknowledging that they are a natural and beautiful part of the journey. Let this be a time of self-appreciation and self-love as you witness the physical transformations that signify the nurturing of a new life.

16

"MY BABY IS A BLESSING, AND I AM GRATEFUL FOR THIS EXPERIENCE"

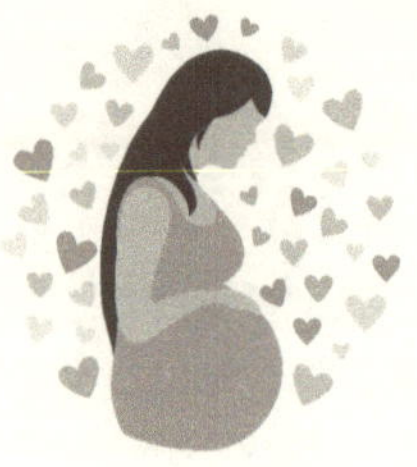

Reflect on the profound gift of motherhood and the blessing of carrying a new life. Express gratitude for the opportunity to nurture and bring forth a precious being into the world. Let this sense of gratitude fill your heart, fostering a deep connection with your baby even before their arrival.

17

"I AM CULTIVATING A DEEP BOND WITH MY UNBORN CHILD"

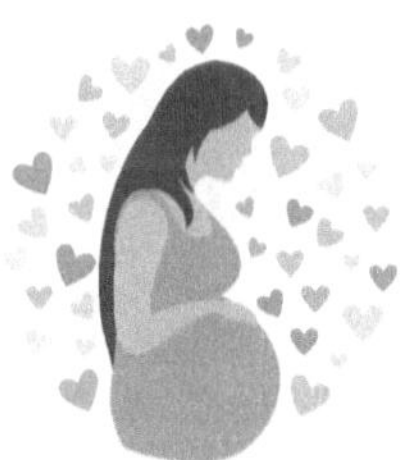

Foster a profound connection with your baby, even before they enter the world. Through your thoughts, actions, and nurturing, you are building a bond that transcends the physical realm. Communicate with your baby, share your hopes and dreams, and let the bond between you grow stronger each day.

18

"I TRUST IN THE WISDOM OF MY BODY TO KNOW WHAT MY BABY NEEDS"

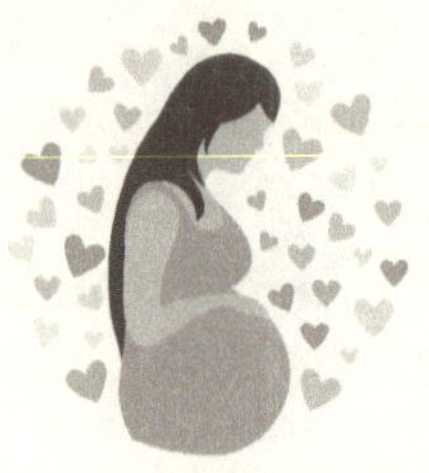

Listen to the intuitive wisdom that emanates from within you. Your body has a deep understanding of what your baby needs for their growth and development. Trust in this intuitive knowledge, and let it guide you in making the best choices for the well-being of your baby.

19

"I AM SURROUNDED BY POSITIVE ENERGY THAT NOURISHES BOTH ME AND MY BABY"

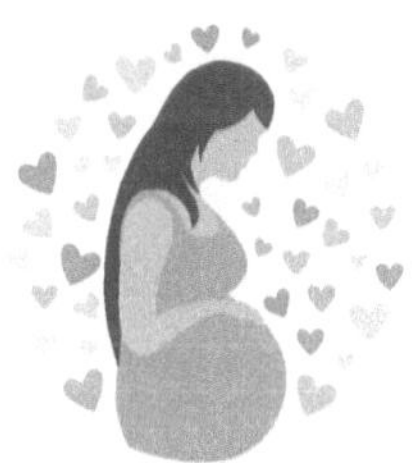

Surround yourself with positivity and optimism. Let the positive energy around you uplift your spirits and nourish both you and your baby. Create a nurturing environment that is filled with joy, peace, and happiness, knowing that this positive atmosphere will have a beneficial impact on your baby's development.

20

"I AM WORTHY OF THIS EXPERIENCE AND CAPABLE OF BEING A GREAT MOTHER"

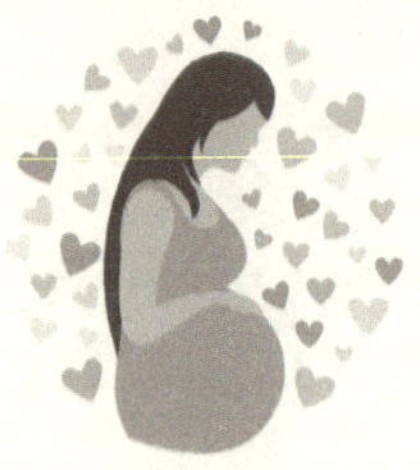

Believe in your inherent worthiness and capability as a mother. Know that you are equipped with the strength, resilience, and love necessary to provide the best possible care for your child. Embrace this journey with confidence, knowing that you are capable of nurturing and guiding your child through life's adventures.

21

"MY BABY IS A SOURCE OF JOY AND HOPE FOR THE FUTURE"

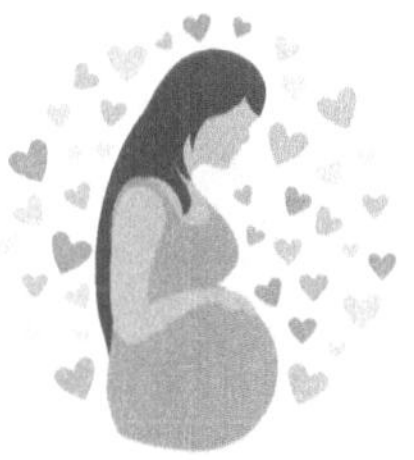

Embrace the profound joy and hope that your baby brings into your life. Let their presence fill your heart with optimism and excitement for the future. Feel the light that their existence brings, illuminating your path and infusing your life with a sense of purpose and meaning.

22

"I AM PATIENT WITH MYSELF AND MY BODY AS IT UNDERGOES THESE CHANGES"

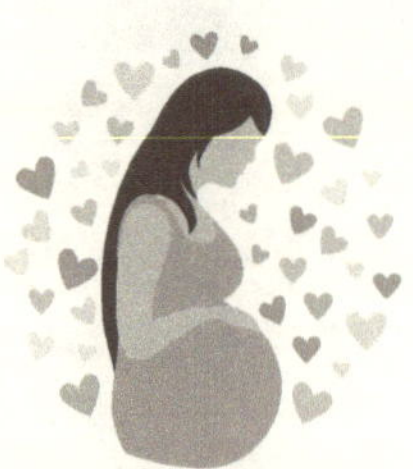

Be gentle with yourself during this transformative journey. Understand that both your body and mind are adapting to the changes that come with pregnancy. Practice patience and self-care, allowing yourself the time and space needed to adjust to these changes and to fully embrace the journey of motherhood.

23

"I AM RELEASING MYSELF FROM ALL FEARS AND EMBRACING THE MIRACLE OF LIFE WITHIN ME"

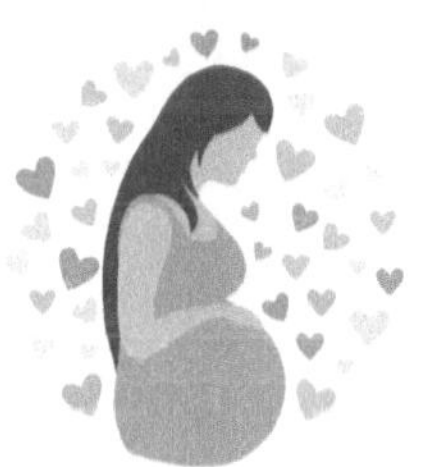

Let go of any fears or anxieties that may cloud your mind. Trust in the natural process of life and the miraculous journey of bringing a new being into the world. Embrace the wonder and beauty of the life growing within you, knowing that you are supported and guided every step of the way.

24

"MY BABY IS SURROUNDED BY AN AURA OF PEACE AND TRANQUILITY"

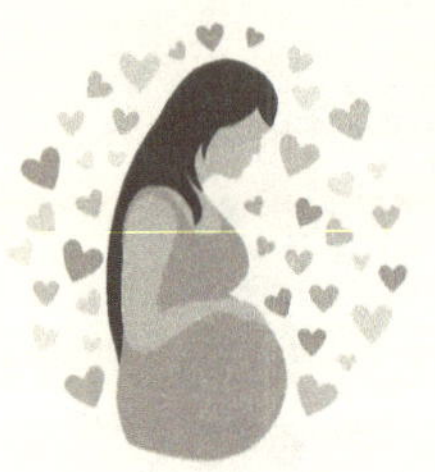

Create a peaceful and serene environment that envelops your baby with a sense of calm and serenity. Let the atmosphere around you be filled with tranquility, fostering a sense of security and peace for your baby. Cultivate a space that is conducive to their growth and well-being, both during pregnancy and beyond.

25

"I AM TAKING CARE OF MYSELF TO ENSURE THE WELL-BEING OF MY BABY"

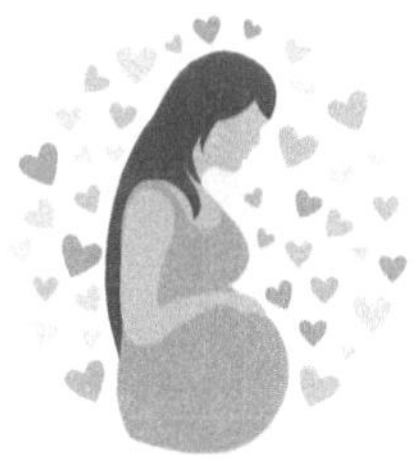

Prioritize your own well-being, knowing that it directly impacts the health and development of your baby. Take the time to rest, eat nourishing foods, and engage in activities that promote your physical and emotional health. By taking care of yourself, you are ensuring a strong foundation for your baby's growth and development.

26

"EACH DAY, I AM BECOMING MORE CONNECTED TO THE LIFE GROWING INSIDE ME"

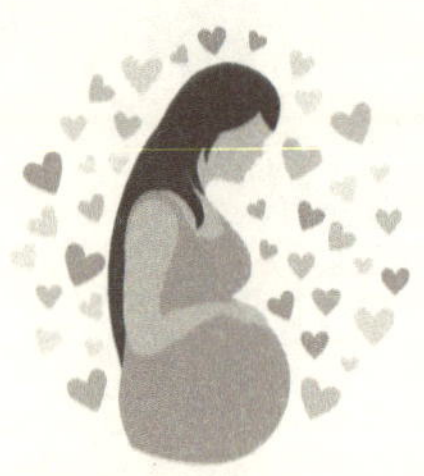

Foster a deep sense of connection with your baby. Allow yourself to be fully present in the journey of pregnancy, nurturing a bond that continues to strengthen with each passing day. Embrace the physical and emotional sensations that come with this connection, knowing that you are sharing a profound experience with the life growing within you.

27

"MY BABY IS A REFLECTION OF LOVE, AND THAT LOVE IS GROWING EVERY DAY"

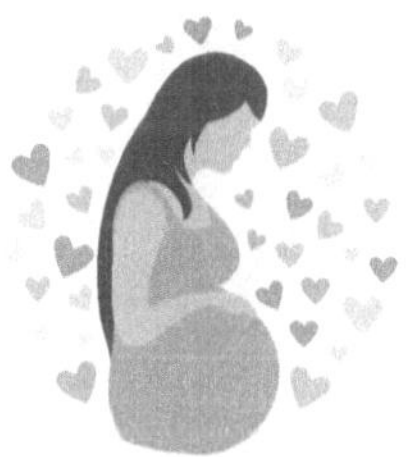

Feel the love expanding within you as your baby grows. Allow this love to flow freely, nurturing your baby's spirit and fostering a strong emotional bond. Embrace the profound connection between you and your baby, knowing that it is a reflection of the boundless love that surrounds and sustains both of you.

28

"I AM ALLOWING MYSELF TO REST AND REJUVENATE FOR THE HEALTH OF MY BABY"

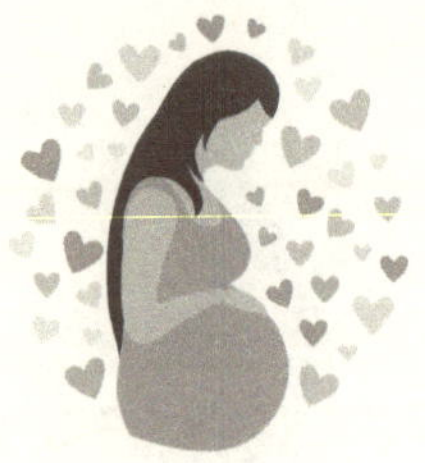

Recognize the importance of rest and rejuvenation during this transformative journey. Give yourself permission to slow down and recharge, knowing that it is essential for your own well-being and that of your baby. Prioritize moments of relaxation and self-care, nurturing your body and mind as you prepare for the arrival of your little one.

29

"I AM CREATING A BEAUTIFUL STORY OF LOVE AND STRENGTH FOR MY CHILD"

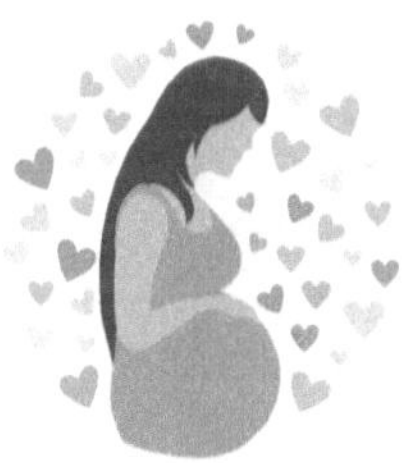

Envision the narrative of love and resilience that you are crafting for your child. Your journey through pregnancy is a testament to the strength and love that will guide your child throughout their life. Embrace the challenges and triumphs as part of this beautiful story, knowing that it will shape the bond you share with your child for years to come.

30

"I AM SURROUNDED BY THE ENERGY OF POSITIVITY AND SERENITY"

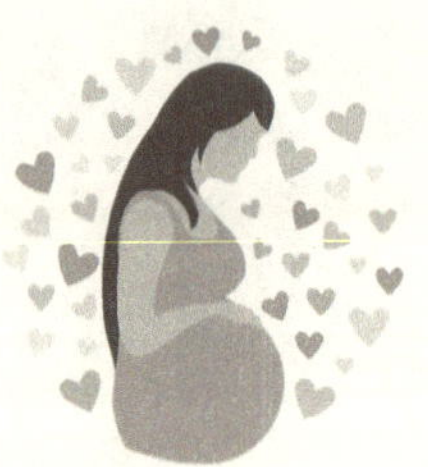

Immerse yourself in an atmosphere of positivity and serenity, allowing these energies to uplift and inspire you. Surround yourself with people and environments that exude optimism and peace, creating a supportive and nurturing space for you and your baby. Let the positive energy around you foster a sense of calm and tranquility, promoting a harmonious and peaceful journey through pregnancy.

31

"I AM RADIATING HAPPINESS AND POSITIVITY FOR MY BABY'S WELL-BEING"

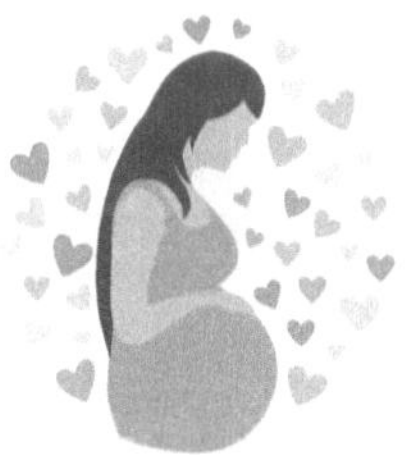

Cultivate a positive and joyful mindset, knowing that your emotional state has a direct impact on your baby's well-being. Let your inner happiness radiate outward, creating an atmosphere of positivity and optimism that envelops both you and your baby. Embrace moments of joy and gratitude, allowing them to resonate within you and nourish your baby's spirit.

32

"I TRUST THE NATURAL PROCESS OF CHILDBIRTH AND EMBRACE IT WITH CONFIDENCE"

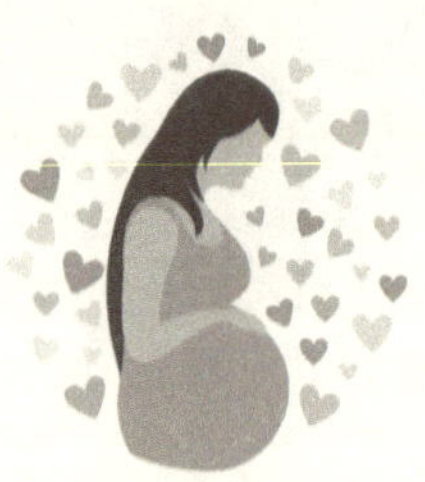

Approach the journey of childbirth with a sense of trust and confidence. Believe in the natural rhythm and wisdom of your body, knowing that it is capable of navigating the process of birth with grace and resilience. Trust in the support and guidance of your healthcare team, and believe in your ability to bring your baby into the world with strength and courage.

33

"I AM GRATEFUL FOR THE SUPPORT OF MY LOVED ONES DURING THIS SPECIAL TIME"

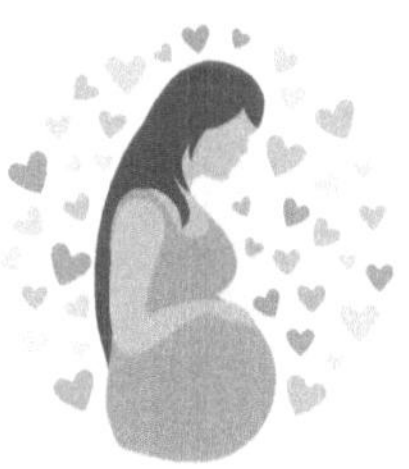

Express gratitude for the unwavering support and love of your family and friends. Acknowledge the importance of their presence in your life, providing you with comfort, guidance, and reassurance throughout your pregnancy journey. Let their support uplift and encourage you, knowing that you are surrounded by a loving community that embraces you and your baby with open arms.

34

"I AM IN TUNE WITH MY BODY AND MY BABY'S NEEDS AT EVERY MOMENT"

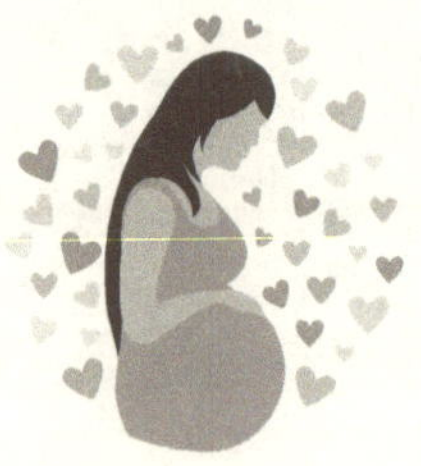

Cultivate a deep awareness of your body and your baby's cues and signals. Listen to the messages that your body conveys and pay attention to the subtle movements and rhythms that your baby communicates. Trust in your intuition and the strong connection you share with your baby, knowing that you are attuned to their needs and well-being.

35

"I AM SENDING LOVE AND PEACE TO MY BABY, NURTURING THEIR SPIRIT AS THEY GROW"

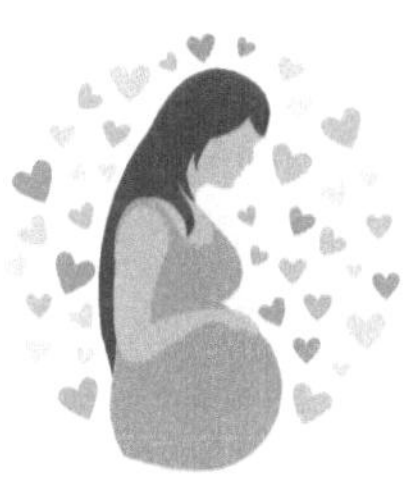

Infuse your thoughts and intentions with love and peace, knowing that your emotional state profoundly impacts your baby's development. Send waves of love and serenity to your baby, fostering a nurturing environment that supports their emotional and spiritual growth. Embrace the power of positive energy, knowing that it nourishes your baby's spirit and fosters a sense of well-being within them.

36

"MY BABY'S ARRIVAL WILL BRING IMMENSE JOY AND FULFILLMENT TO MY LIFE"

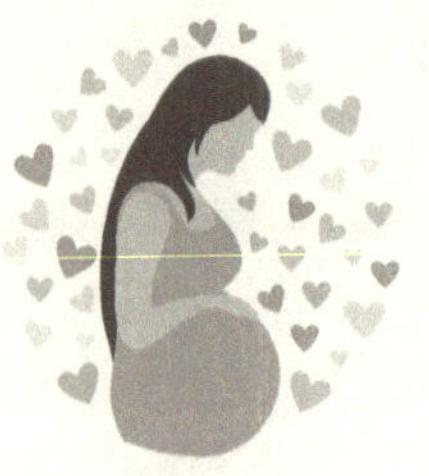

Anticipate the profound joy and fulfillment that your baby's arrival will bring into your life. Embrace the excitement and happiness that come with the prospect of meeting your little one for the first time. Let the anticipation of their arrival fill your heart with a sense of wonder and anticipation, knowing that their presence will enrich your life in immeasurable ways.

37

"MY BABY IS A SYMBOL OF HOPE AND NEW BEGINNINGS IN MY LIFE"

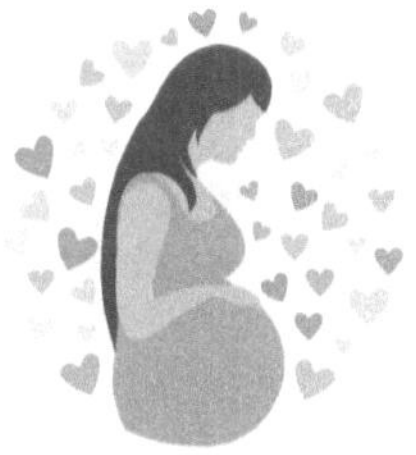

Embrace the symbolism of your baby as a beacon of hope and new beginnings. Allow their impending arrival to signify a fresh chapter in your life, filled with optimism and promise. Let the anticipation of their birth ignite a sense of hope and renewal within you, inspiring you to embrace the future with a newfound sense of purpose and determination.

38

"I AM CREATING A LOVING AND NURTURING ENVIRONMENT FOR MY CHILD TO THRIVE"

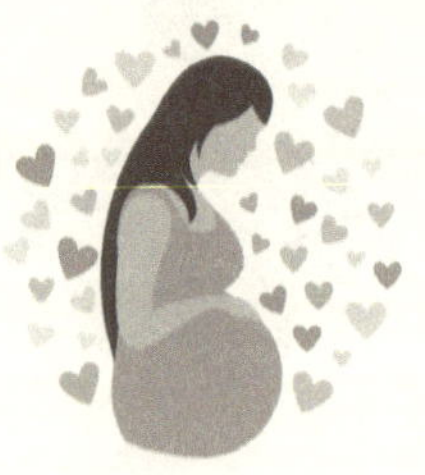

Foster a loving and nurturing environment that promotes your child's growth and well-being. Cultivate a space filled with love, compassion, and understanding, laying the foundation for a harmonious and supportive upbringing. Let your home be a sanctuary of warmth and security, nurturing your child's physical, emotional, and spiritual development.

39

"I AM CALM AND PREPARED FOR THE BEAUTIFUL JOURNEY OF CHILDBIRTH"

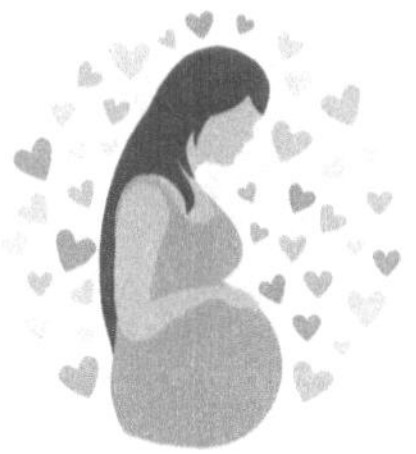

Approach the journey of childbirth with a sense of inner calm and preparedness. Embrace the transformative experience with a composed and peaceful mindset, knowing that you have the strength and resilience to navigate this process with grace and courage. Cultivate a sense of serenity and composure, allowing it to guide you through the miraculous journey of bringing your baby into the world.

40

"I TRUST MY INTUITION IN MAKING THE BEST DECISIONS FOR MY BABY'S WELL-BEING"

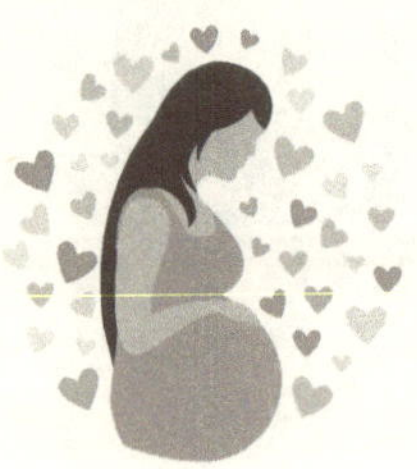

Embrace the wisdom that emanates from your intuition, knowing that it serves as a guiding light in making decisions for your baby's well-being. Trust in your instincts and inner knowing, allowing them to lead you toward choices that promote the health and happiness of your child. Believe in the strength of your maternal intuition, knowing that it is a powerful tool in nurturing and caring for your baby.

41

"I AM ACCEPTING THE SUPPORT AND ASSISTANCE OFFERED TO ME WITH GRATITUDE"

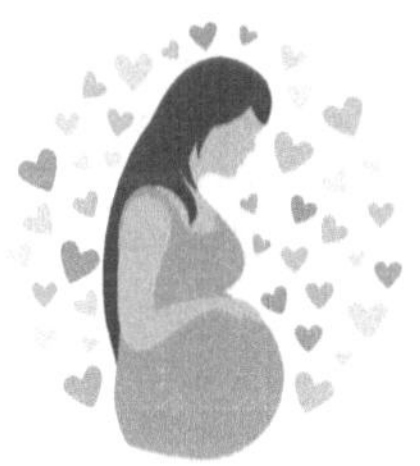

Embrace the support and assistance extended to you with open arms and a grateful heart. Accept the love and care that others offer, knowing that it is a testament to the strong bonds of community and connection. Express gratitude for the helping hands and comforting words that uplift and encourage you, knowing that you are not alone on this journey.

42

"I AM ENVISIONING A SMOOTH AND PEACEFUL CHILDBIRTH FOR MYSELF AND MY BABY"

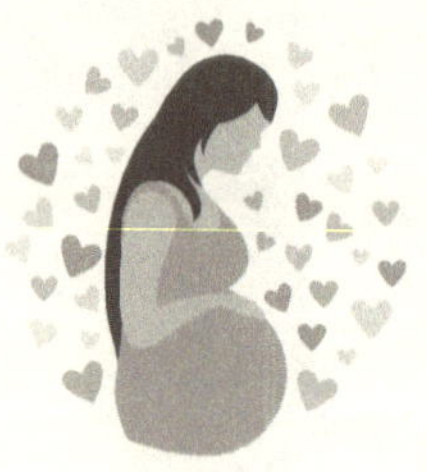

Visualize a childbirth experience that is smooth, peaceful, and filled with serenity. Paint a picture of tranquility and calmness that envelops you and your baby, creating an atmosphere of relaxation and ease. Let this visualization guide your thoughts and intentions, fostering a sense of confidence and assurance as you approach the miraculous moment of bringing your baby into the world.

43

"I AM RESILIENT AND CAPABLE OF HANDLING THE CHALLENGES OF MOTHERHOOD"

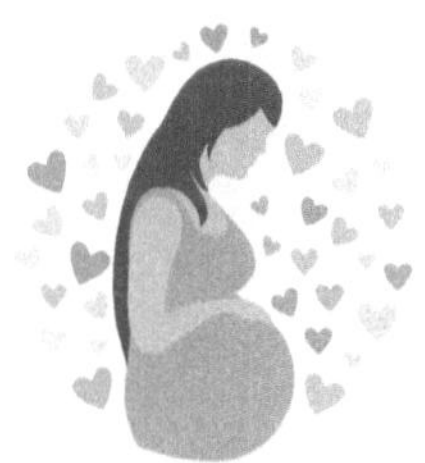

Embrace your inner resilience and strength as you prepare to embark on the journey of motherhood. Recognize the challenges that may arise and trust in your ability to navigate them with grace and fortitude. Believe in your capacity to adapt and grow, knowing that each challenge presents an opportunity for learning and personal development.

44

"MY BABY IS A SYMBOL OF HOPE AND THE FUTURE, BRINGING LIGHT INTO MY LIFE"

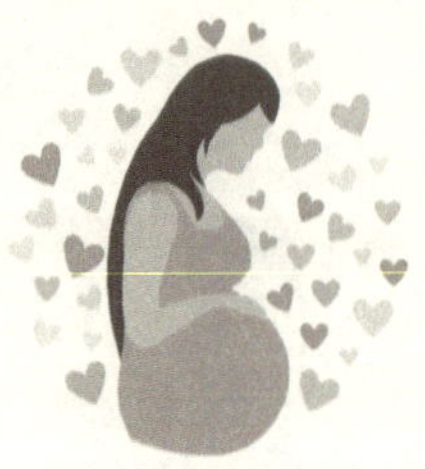

Embrace the symbolism of your baby as a beacon of hope and a representation of the future. Let their impending arrival fill your life with light and optimism, igniting a sense of purpose and determination within you. Embrace the joy and anticipation that come with the prospect of welcoming a new life, knowing that your baby's presence signifies a bright and promising future ahead.

45

"MY BABY IS A SOURCE OF WONDER AND AMAZEMENT, BRINGING JOY TO MY LIFE"

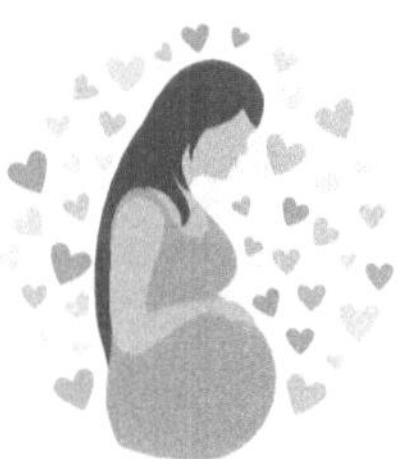

Embrace the wonder and amazement that your baby brings into your life. Allow their presence to fill your heart with boundless joy and happiness, knowing that they are a precious gift that enriches your world. Let the magic of their existence inspire you to see the world with fresh eyes, fostering a sense of wonder and curiosity that you can share with your child as they grow.

46

"I AM ALLOWING MYSELF TO FULLY EXPERIENCE THE JOYS OF PREGNANCY"

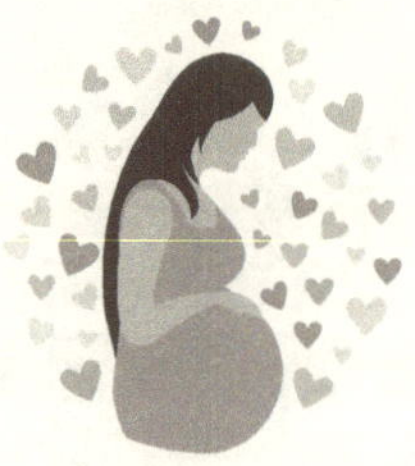

Embrace the joys and wonders that come with the journey of pregnancy. Allow yourself to fully immerse in the experience, savoring every moment and milestone. Cherish the sensations and emotions that accompany this transformative journey, knowing that each experience contributes to the profound connection you share with your baby.

47

"I AM CREATING A STRONG AND UNBREAKABLE BOND WITH MY BABY"

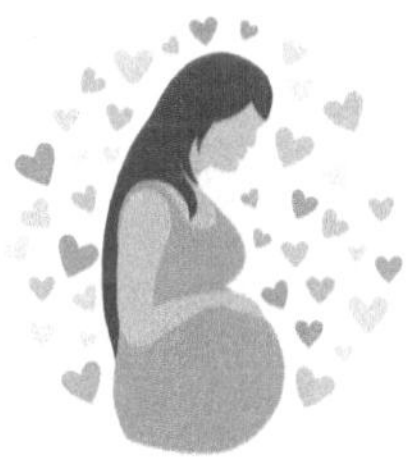

Foster a deep and unbreakable bond with your baby, establishing a connection that transcends the physical realm. Engage in activities that promote bonding and communication, nurturing a relationship that is built on love, trust, and understanding. Cultivate a strong foundation for your mother-child relationship, knowing that it will serve as a source of support and guidance for both of you in the years to come.

48

"MY BABY'S HEALTH AND WELL-BEING ARE MY TOP PRIORITIES, AND I AM TAKING CARE OF BOTH OF US"

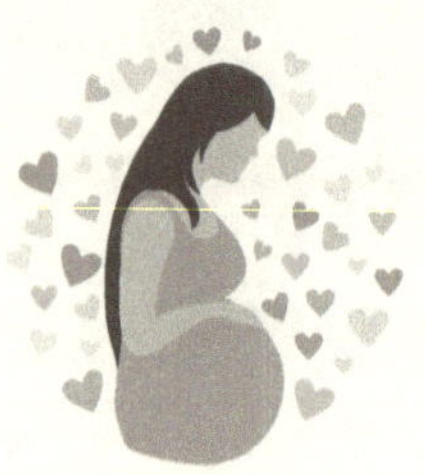

Prioritize the health and well-being of both yourself and your baby. Make conscious choices that promote physical and emotional wellness, ensuring that you are both nourished and supported throughout the pregnancy journey. Embrace a holistic approach to self-care, knowing that your well-being directly impacts your baby's health and development.

49

"I AM SURROUNDED BY AN ABUNDANCE OF LOVE AND POSITIVITY FOR MY GROWING FAMILY"

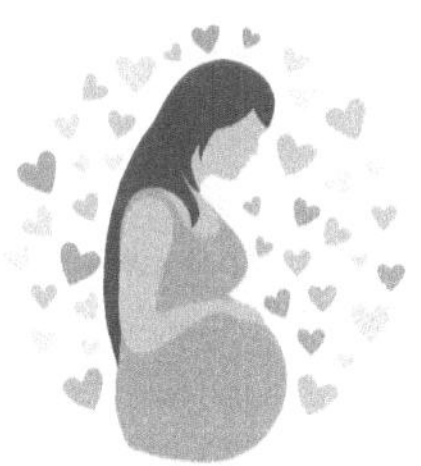

Embrace the abundance of love and positivity that surrounds you and your growing family. Let the bonds of love and support strengthen and flourish, creating a nurturing and uplifting environment for you and your baby. Bask in the warmth and affection of your loved ones, knowing that their presence enriches your life and enhances the journey of motherhood.

50

"MY BABY IS A REFLECTION OF THE LOVE AND CARE I PROVIDE DURING THIS JOURNEY"

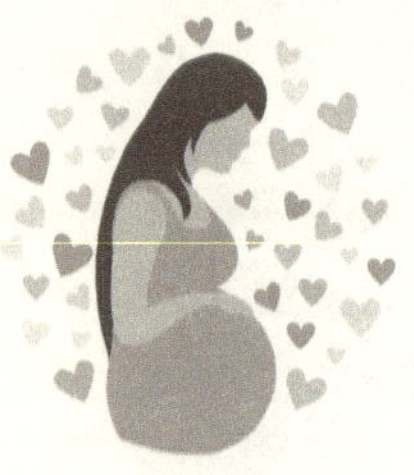

Recognize the profound influence of your love and care on your baby's well-being and development. Understand that your nurturing presence shapes their early experiences, fostering a sense of security and trust that will resonate throughout their life. Embrace the opportunity to provide a nurturing and loving environment, knowing that your actions and intentions have a lasting impact on your baby's emotional and cognitive development.

51

"I AM HAVING A NORMAL BABY, EVERY ORGANS AND CELLS OF MY BABY ARE NORMAL AND EXCELLENT"

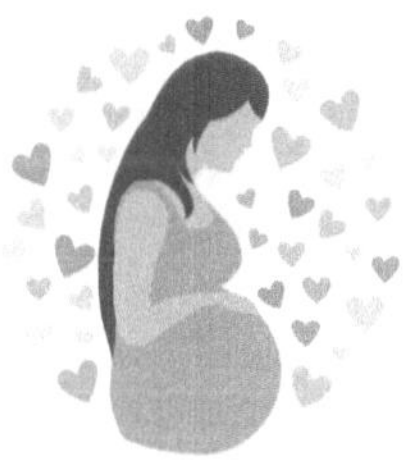

The greatest fear of a mother is the 'what ifs'. It's not a matter of whether your baby is a boy or a girl. Sometimes when you think about your baby or when you see anything that is abnormal, you fear what if that happen to your baby. Stop fearing, instead visualize seeing your baby completely normal with every organs and cells - a completely healthy baby.

52

"I AM CONNECTED TO THE GENERATIONS OF MOTHERS WHO HAVE COME BEFORE ME"

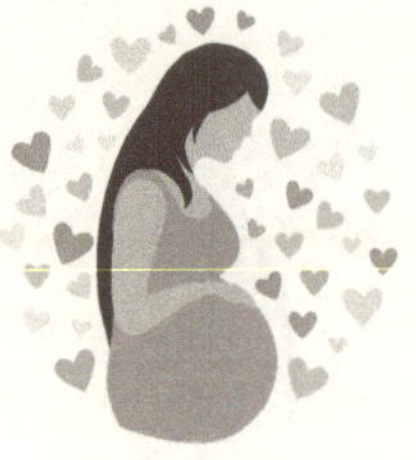

Acknowledge the deep-rooted connection you share with the generations of mothers who have walked this path before you. Draw strength and inspiration from the collective wisdom and experience of these women, knowing that you are part of a lineage of resilience and nurturing. Embrace the lessons and legacies passed down through generations, allowing them to guide and support you as you navigate the journey of motherhood.

These affirmations are a powerful reminder of your strength and potential in becoming a good mother. Speak to yourself daily, and let them serve as a source of motivation to become the best version of yourself.

May you have a normal, healthy, strong, and beautiful baby. May you be the best Mom you could ever be!

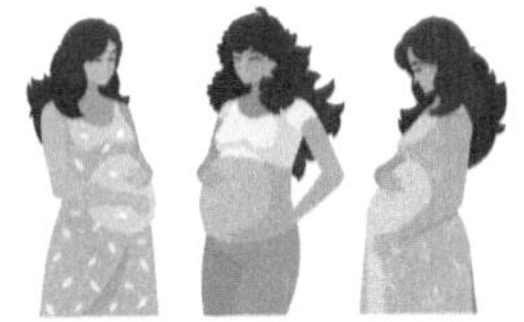

About The Author:

M Ngaihlian is a nurse by profession and a mother of two beautiful angels. Her passion for writing rekindles as she re-dedicated her life to be a voice, a shoulder to cry on, a helping hand for those downtrodden, outcast, and ignored people in society, and proclaim the love of God and His unfailing mercy and grace. She can be found online at pourbin.com.

www.ingramcontent.com/pod-product-compliance
Lightning Source LLC
Chambersburg PA
CBHW031424250726
48656CB00002B/815